# Lean Green Smoothie Machine

# 25 Delicious Weight Loss and Detox Recipes

*By Clark Moraign*

# Table of Contents

# Introduction

First, I want to thank you for purchasing Lean Green Smoothie Machine. This book is for anyone who is looking to lose weight or maintain their current weight, it is also for anyone who would like to detox their bodies. Any weight loss program should always include physical activity and detoxing your body. In fact just increasing your physical activity and drink water will help to detox your body, because physical movement like lifting weights and cardio, as in running will speed up your metabolism which will also increase fat lose My Name is Clark Moraign and I have a passion for working out and staying healthy and if you are looking for delicious weight loss and detox smoothie recipes then this is the right book for you. In side this book you will find, first smoothie recipes that will help you to lose weight or maintain your desired weight. You will find detox recipes in here, quite a few in fact, there are a total of 25 combined weight loss and detox recipes. I also threw in 8 bonus recipes for a total of 33 different recipes. Also if you are looking for a great Smoothie machine check out this one NUTRIBULLET, I personally use it and you can get in on Amazon,

If you like to work out and are looking for some recipes with high quality proteins in them. Check out my other book. Lean Muscle Building Recipes.

Enjoy the recipes and do share with your family and friends.

# 1. Cherry Raspberry Breakfast

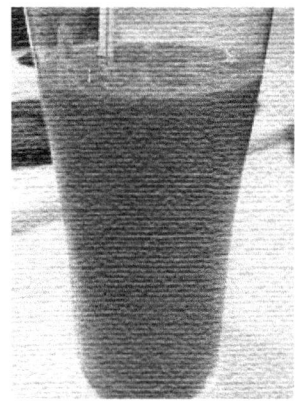

Cherry Raspberry Breakfast

Ingredients

1 cup frozen unsweetened raspberries
3/4 cup chilled unsweetened almond or rice milk
1/4 cup frozen pitted unsweetened cherries or raspberries
1 1/2 Tbsps. honey
2 tsp finely grated fresh ginger
1 tsp ground flaxseed
1-2 tsp fresh lemon juice

Blend until smooth.

Serves 2

# 2. Berry Blast

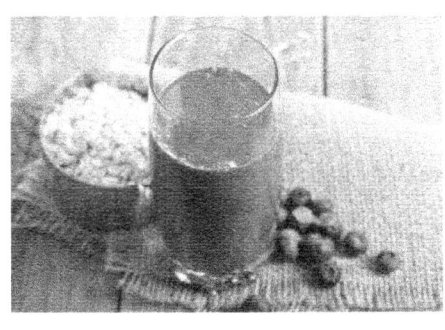

Berry Blast

Ingredients

1 1/2 cups mixed berries, blueberries, raspberries, blackberries
1/2 cup Coconut Milk
1 cup Purified Water

1/8 cup rolled oats
Blend until smooth.

Serves 2

# 3. Goji and Strawberry Smoothie

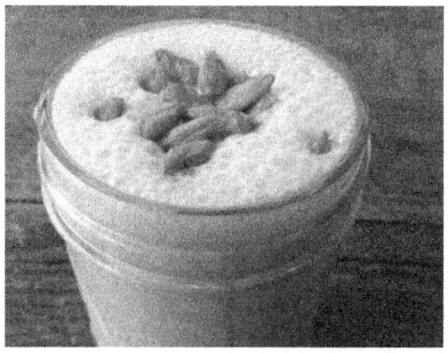

Goji and Strawberry Smoothie

Ingredients

1 cup of coconut kefir water
1 frozen banana
¼ cup frozen strawberries (a some ice if strawberries and not frozen)
3 Tbsps. Goji berries

Blend until Smooth

Serves 1

# 4. Ginger's Blueberries and Banana Smoothie

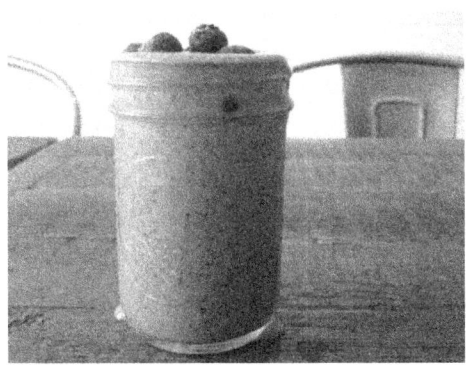

Ginger's Blueberries and Banana Smoothie

Ingredients

1 cup almond milk, or any type of milk you like.
¼ cup blueberries
1 frozen banana (add ice if banana is not frozen)
3 Tbsps. ginger juice

Blend until smooth

Serves 1

# 5. Mango and Vanilla yogurt Smoothie

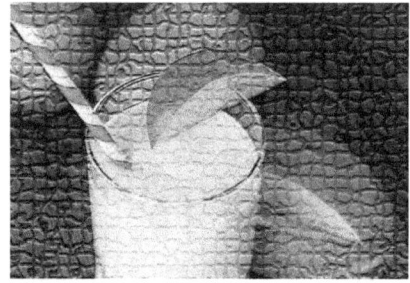

Mango and Vanilla yogurt Smoothie

Ingredients

¼ cup mango cubes
¼ cup mashed ripe avocado (MUFA)
½ cup mango juice
¼ cup fat-free vanilla yogurt
1 Tbsps. freshly squeezed lime juice
1 Tbsps. sugar
6 ice cubes

Blend until smooth

Serves 1

# 6. Georgia Peach Smoothie

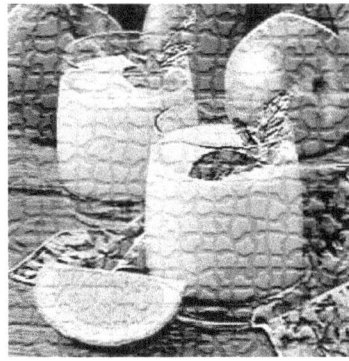

Georgia Peach Smoothie

Ingredients

1 cup skim milk
1 cup frozen unsweetened peaches
2 tsp cold-pressed organic flaxseed oil

Blend until smooth pour into a glass then stir in flaxseed oil.

Serves 1

# 7. Tropical Breeze Smoothie

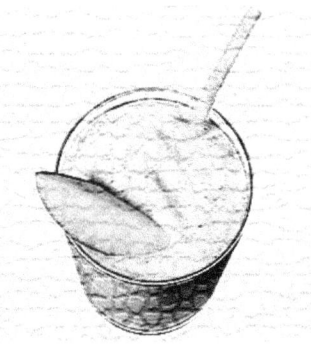

Tropical Breeze Smoothie

Ingredients

6 ounces plain nonfat Greek yogurt
1/2 cup fresh or frozen mango chunks
1/2 cup fresh pineapple chunks
1 frozen banana, chopped
2 tablespoons ground flaxseed

Blend until smooth, pout in to glasses and add flaxseed

Serves 1

# 8. Honeydew and Kiwi Smoothie

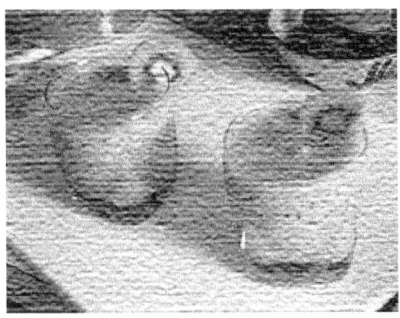

Honeydew and Kiwi Smoothie

Ingredients

2 cups of honeydew, cubed
1 Granny Smith apple, chopped
1 kiwi fruit, peeled and chopped
2 tablespoons of sugar
1 tablespoon of lemon juice
1 cup of ice cubes

Directions

Place the honeydew, kiwi, apple, sugar, and lemon juice into the blender and blend until it's smooth. Then add the ice cubes and blend until the mixture is slushy.

Serves 2

# 9. Pineapple Smoothie

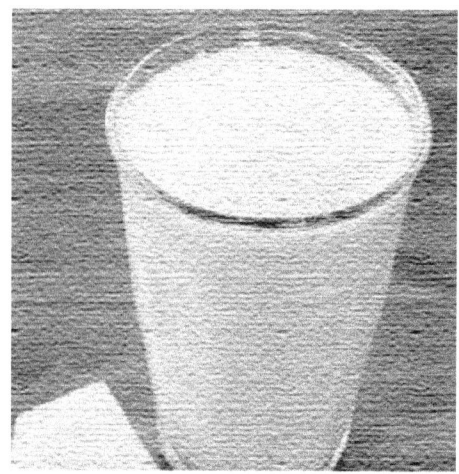

Pineapple Smoothie

Ingredients

1 of cup skim milk
4 ounces canned pineapple chunks, with the juice
1 tablespoon of flaxseed oil
6 ice cubes

Blend until smooth, then pour into glass and add flaxseed oil

Serves 1

# 10. Pomegranate Smoothie

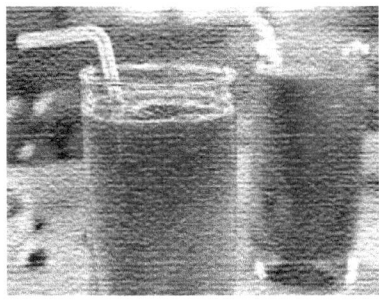

Pomegranate Smoothie

Ingredients

1 ½ cups of frozen berries – again you can use any berries that you want or mix them up
1 cup pomegranate juice – unsweetened1 pomegranate
1 ounce whey protein powder
1 tablespoon honey


Blend until smooth

Serves 1

# 11. Watermelon Smoothie

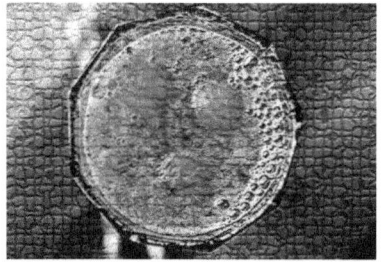

Watermelon Smoothie

Ingredients

6 cups of seedless watermelon, chopped
1 cup of lemon sherbet, non-fat milk, or low-fat vanilla yogurt
12 ice cubes

Directions

Put half the watermelon in the blender and blend until smooth,
Then add half of the ice and sherbet; blend until smooth.
Repeat the process with the rest of the ingredients.

Serves 4

# 12. Mango and Kale

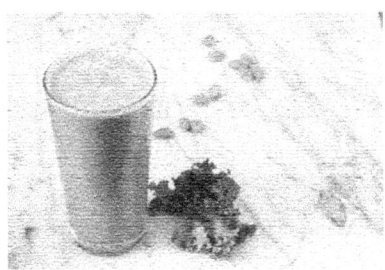

Mango and Kale

Ingredients

1¼ cups frozen cubed mango
1¼ cups chopped kale leaves
2 medium ribs celery, chopped
1 cup chilled fresh tangerine or orange juice
¼ cup chopped flat-leaf parsley
¼ cup chopped fresh mint

Blend until smooth.

Serves 2

# 13. Green Glow Smoothie

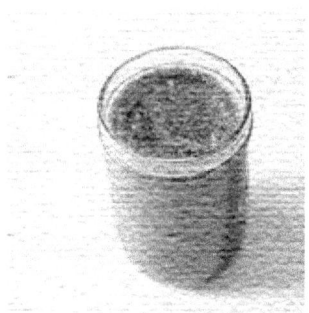

Green Glow Smoothie.

Ingredients

1 1/2 cups water
1 head organic romaine lettuce, chopped
3 to 4 stalks organic celery
1/2 head of a large bunch or 3/4 of a small bunch of spinach
1 organic apple, cored and chopped
1 organic pear, cored and chopped
1 organic banana
Juice of 1/2 fresh organic lemon
1/3 bunch organic cilantro
1/3 bunch organic parsley

DIRECTIONS

In a blender, add water.
Add chopped head of romaine. Blend at a low speed until smooth.
Add spinach, celery, apple, and pear, and blend at high speed.
Add cilantro and parsley.
Finish with banana and lemon.

Serves 2

# 14. Super Green Juice Detox

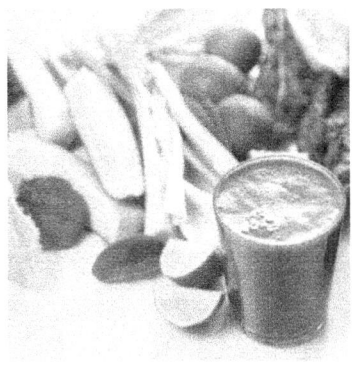

Super Green Juice Detox

Ingredients

Ingredients
2 celery stalks
1 small cucumber,
Chopped 2 kale leaves
1 handful spinach
Handful of fresh parsley 1 lemon peeled
1 apple, seeded, cored and chopped

Directions

If using a juicer, add all the above ingredients.
If using a blender, add all the above ingredients
With 1 cup chilled water. Blend until smooth.

Serves 2

# 15. Citrus Detox Water

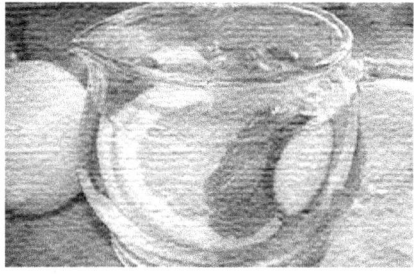

Citrus Detox Water

Ingredients

Ingredients
½ gallon purified water
½ lemon, sliced
½ lime, sliced
½ grapefruit, sliced
1 cup cucumber, sliced
1 tsp ginger, sliced (add more if you like)
A small handful of peppermint leaves

Directions

Place all the ingredients in a large picture, add ice (optional).
Place in the fridge for 2 hours and drink. If left in the fridge longer then 24 hours throw out.

# 16. Morning Glory

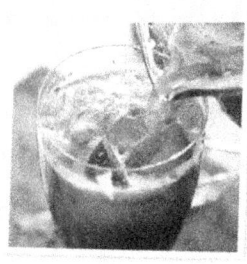

Morning Glory

Ingredients

1 large cucumber
A handful of kale
A handful of romaine
3 stalks celery
1 large broccoli stem
1 green apple, quartered
½ peeled lemon, quartered


JUICE all ingredients.
If using a blender, add 1 cup of water

Serves 2

# 17. The Spicy Sicilian

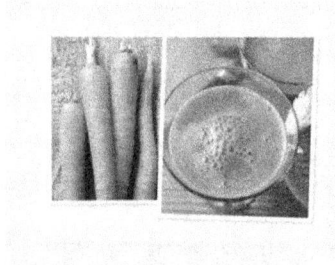

The Spicy Sicilian

Ingredients

6 carrots
3 large tomatoes
2 red bell peppers
4 cloves garlic
4 stalks celery
1 cup watercress
1 cup loosely packed spinach
1 red jalapeño, seeded (if you like seeds)

Directions

Juice all ingredients
If using a blender add 1 cup of water

Serves 1

# 18. The Blueberry Lemon

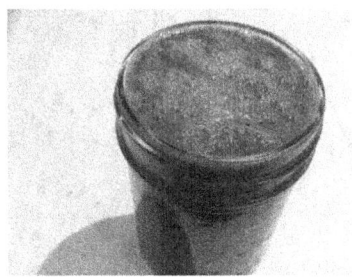

The Blueberry Lemon

Ingredients

1 cup alkaline water
¼ cup organic blueberries
1 organic lemon (whole).

BLEND all ingredients.

Serves 1

# 19. Apple Mint Berry Detox

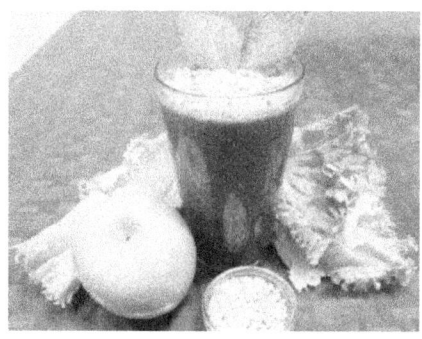

Apple Mint Berry Detox

Ingredients

½ green apple
2 tablespoons of Manitoba Harvest Hemp Hearts
8 fresh mint leaves
3-4 leaves of organic green leaf lettuce
¼ cup organic fresh or frozen berry blend
8-12 oz. pure water

Blend until smooth

Serves 1-2

# 20. Sensual Morning Detox

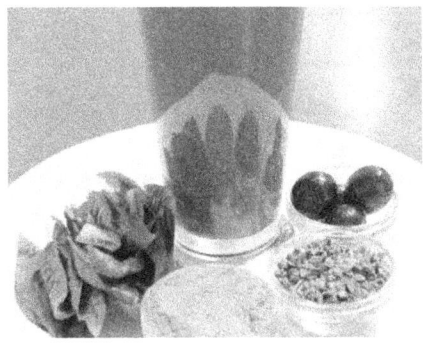

Sensual Morning Detox

Ingredients

1 tablespoon of cacao powder
2 tablespoons of hemp seeds
4-5 red endive leaves
Pinch of green stevia
¼ cup of organic fresh or frozen dark red cherries
8-12 oz. pure water

Blend until smooth

Serves 1-2

# 21. March Detox Smoothie

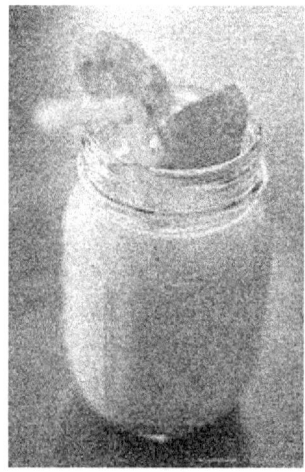

March Detox Smoothie

Ingredients

Ingredients
1 cup green tea, chilled
1 cup loosely packed cilantro
1 cup loosely packed organic baby kale
1 cup cucumber
1 cup pineapple
 Juice of 1 lemon
1 tablespoon fresh ginger, grated
½ avocado


Blend until smooth.

Serves 1

# 22. Mean Green Detox Smoothie

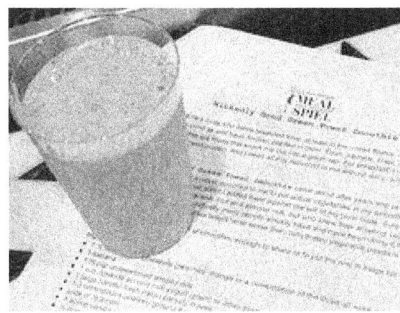

Mean Green Detox Smoothie

Ingredients

3 cups organic spinach
1 cup frozen mixed berries
1 cup frozen mango or peach
1 frozen banana
1 tablespoon spiraling
1 tablespoon maple syrup
1 tablespoon coconut oil
2 tablespoon chia seeds
2 cups almond milk
Small handful of fresh parsley or mint
Pomegranate seeds for topping

Blend until Smooth

Serves 2

# 23. Super Broccoli Orange Apple Protector

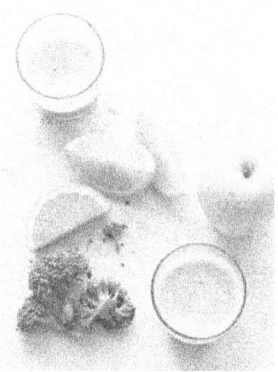

Super Broccoli Orange Apple Protector

Ingredients

2 cups chopped broccoli, stems and florets
2 large oranges, peeled and seeded
1 large apple, cored

First, juice the broccoli, oranges, and apple, then
Run the pulp through again to extract as much liquid as possible.
If using a blender add 1 cup of water.

Serves 2

# 24. Turmeric Ginger Honey Bomb

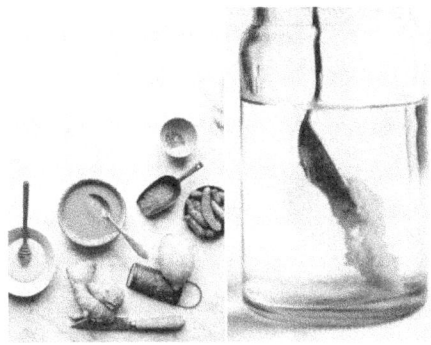

Turmeric Ginger Honey Bomb

Ingredients


1/2 cup Organic Honey
2-4 tbsp. freshly grated or ground ginger.
2 tsp grated or ground turmeric
1 organic untaxed lemon, freshly grated zest
2 pinches ground black pepper

Stir together all ingredients in a bowl. You will only be adding a few teaspoons to a cup of water. Store the Turmeric Ginger Honey Bomb in a glass container.

Boil a cup of water and let slightly cool, stir in a few teaspoons of the Turmeric Ginger Honey Bomb mixture and drink.
If you like you could also at a few teaspoons to your favorite hot tea.

Makes about 1/2 cup

# 25. Chili and Blood Orange Juice

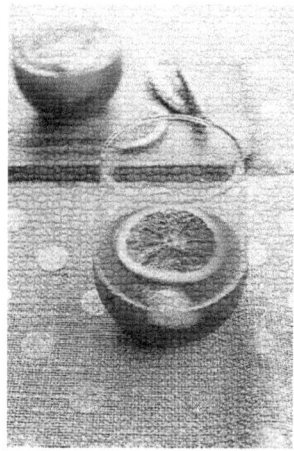

Chili and Blood Orange Juice

Ingredients

 2 Serrano Chili
6 Blood Oranges
Agave Nectar


PREPARATION
1. Juice blood oranges. If using a blender add 1 cup of water.
2. Dice serrano chilies, soak Chilies in the juice for 24 hours.
3. Strain juice, removing all the chili.
4. Add agave for additional sweetening.

Serves 2

# 26. Banana and Peanut Butter Smoothie

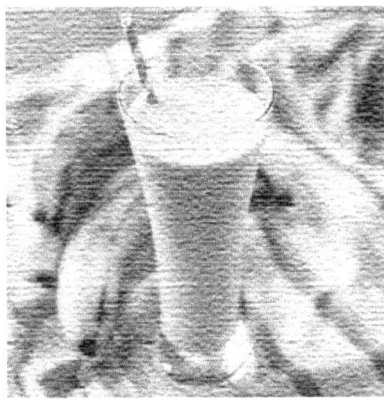

Banana and Peanut Butter Smoothie

Ingredients

½ c fat-free milk
½ c fat-free plain yogurt
2 Tbsps. creamy natural unsalted peanut butter
¼ very ripe banana
1 Tbsps. honey
4 ice cubes

Blend until smooth

Serves 1

# 27. Vanilla Yogurt and Blueberry Smoothie

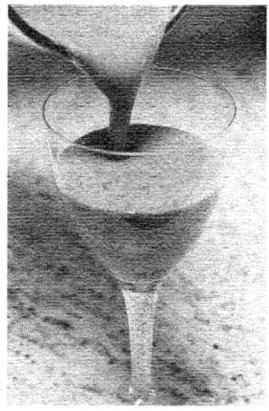

Vanilla Yogurt and Blueberry Smoothie

Ingredients

1 cup skim or soy milk
6 oz. vanilla yogurt
1 cup fresh blueberries
 A few ice cubes (if your blueberries are not frozen)
1 Tbsps. flaxseed oil

Blend milk, yogurt, and fresh blueberries (frozen blueberries or us ice)
When done blending until smooth pour into a glass then stir in flaxseed oil.

Serves 1

# 28. Raspberry Chocolate Smoothie

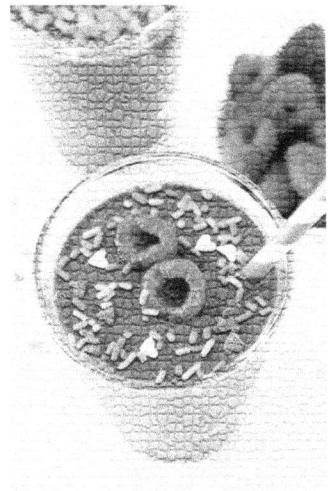

Raspberry Chocolate Smoothie

Ingredients

½ cup skim or soy milk
6 oz. vanilla yogurt
¼ cup chocolate chips
1 cup fresh raspberries
Handful of ice OR 1 cup frozen raspberries

Blend until smooth

Serves 1

# 29. Sweet Spinach and Yogurt Smoothie

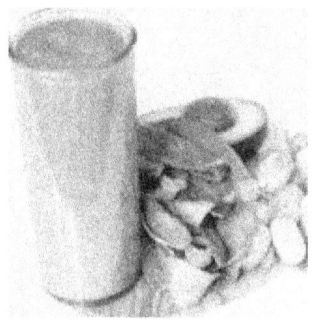

Sweet Spinach and Yogurt Smoothie

Ingredients

6 ounces plain nonfat Greek yogurt
2 cups spinach leaves, packed
1 ripe pear, peeled, cored, and chopped
15 green or red grapes
2 tablespoons chopped avocado
1 to 2 tablespoons freshly squeezed lime juice

Blend until smooth

Serves 2

# 30. Mocha Madness Smoothie

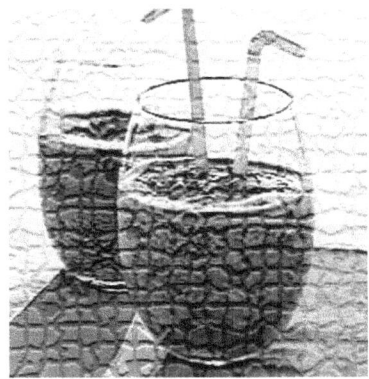

Mocha Madness Smoothie

Ingredients

4 small ice cubes
1/2 cup of low-fat vanilla frozen #yogurt
1 shot of espresso
2 teaspoons of cocoa powder

Blend until smooth

Serves 1

# 31. Pecan Pie Apple Smoothie

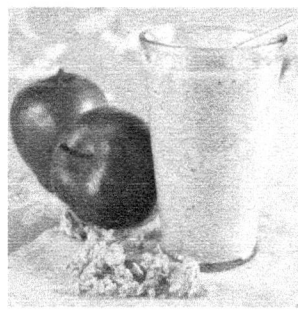

Pecan Pie Apple Smoothie

Ingredients

An apple with the skin left on
¼ unsalted pecans1 cup
1 cup unsweetened coconut milk
3 to 4 ice cubes
1 tablespoons vanilla protein powder
1 tablespoon coconut butter
A dash of cinnamon to taste
A dash of nutmeg
Just a few drops of stevia liquid or another sweetener to taste

Blend until smooth

Serves 2

# 32. Banana Coconut Smoothie

Banana Coconut Smoothie

Ingredients

8 ounces of coconut milk
2 eggs
1 tablespoon Extra Virgin coconut oil
1 frozen banana
¼ cup berries (any berries)

Blend until smooth

Serves 1

# 33. The Chubby Chaser Juice

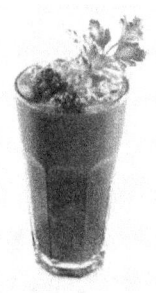

The Chubby Chaser Juice

Ingredients

1 medium organic red beet
3 medium organic carrots
1 organic radish
2 organic garlic cloves
Large handful of organic parsley

Juice and serve, if you are using a blender add 1 cup of water

Serves 1

# Conclusion

Thanks again for downloading Lean Green Smoothie Machine. I'm in the process of writing more recipe and other health and fitness books. You may also be interested in my other books,

Lean Muscle Building Recipes.

Burn Fat Build Muscle Beastmode

A little history about me. Ever since I was a kid growing up in Texas, I have had a passion for working out and staying fit. I played Football in High School and then joined the United States Army where I became an Infantry Soldier. As an 11-Bravo part of my job was to be in and stay in top physical condition, 32 Years after joining the Army at the age of 18, my passion is still working out and staying fit and I plan to share what I know with you and others.

So I am starting a free book club, which means whenever I launch a new book I will make it free for you to download via Amazon's Kindle Book Store. If you are interested in joining my free book club, SIGN UP HERE, I will send you updates and information about upcoming books and products.

If you enjoyed this book, would you please leave a review for this book on Amazon? It'd be greatly appreciated!

Finally, if you find any problems or areas that you feel could be better in this book, please let me know so that I can address them. Again, you can reach me at readdragonpublishing@gmail.com

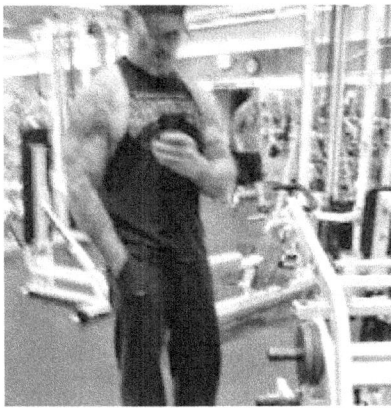

Thank you
Clark Moraign